Harry and C
Queensland,
Made Easy was a word-of-mouth success
(naturally!) before it was taken on by a
publisher.

Harry and Caddie are happy to receive any
feedback from readers. You can send your
comments, suggestions and reactions to them
at <u>HarryCaddie@bigpond.com</u>

MOUTH MUSIC MADE EASY

How to drive her wild with pleasure

HARRY and CADDIE YOUNGBERRY

CORGI BOOKS

MOUTH MUSIC MADE EASY
A CORGI BOOK : 0 552 14973 X

Originally published in Australia by Random House Australia
(Pty) Ltd.
First publication in Great Britain

PRINTING HISTORY
Corgi edition published 2002

1 3 5 7 9 10 8 6 4 2

Copyright © W.D. Harry Youngberry 2001

The right of Harry and Caddie Youngberry to be identified as
the authors of this work has been asserted in accordance with
sections 77 and 78 of the Copyright Designs and Patents Act
1988.

Set in 12/13pt Garamond 3 by
Phoenix Typesetting, Burley-in-Wharfedale, West Yorkshire.

Corgi Books are published by Transworld Publishers,
61–63 Uxbridge Road, London W5 5SA,
a division of The Random House Group Ltd,
in Australia by Random House Australia (Pty) Ltd,
20 Alfred Street, Milsons Point, Sydney, NSW 2061, Australia,
in New Zealand by Random House New Zealand Ltd,
18 Poland Road, Glenfield, Auckland 10, New Zealand
and in South Africa by Random House (Pty) Ltd,
Endulini, 5a Jubilee Road, Parktown 2193, South Africa.

Printed and bound in Great Britain by
Clays Ltd, St Ives plc.

MOUTH MUSIC
MADE EASY

Foreword

There is a running joke around our house where my lovely Caddie, in her glorious drifting *aftergasm*, reckons she should rent me out, or at least my tongue. The sums of money Caddie estimates I could command would keep us in luxury if I 'worked' only one hour a week.

Fortunately (or unfortunately) this is just our little joke and it's going to stay that way. But that doesn't mean this special skill of mine should stay a secret.

One day, in the midst of pleasuring Caddie with said rentable tongue, I realized that the viable alternative was to write a book about this curious and rewarding occupation. Inspiration comes at the damnedest times, doesn't it?

If I could write about other things, why not this? But how do I elicit such clitoral satisfaction, I wondered. How do I *do* it? But then how do I drive a

car, ride a bike, walk down the street,
breathe the air? I'd forgotten how to do
it, I just *did*.

After hours of research (I will not say
long hours because I really enjoyed the
research – so did Caddie) this small book
emerged. Whether it contains anything
'new' is beside the point. The Egyptians
were doing sex this way before they
built the pyramids, and so were a lot
of other people.

What I hope this book will do for you
is help you bring out your own natural
talents. You may need a little practice.
I certainly didn't get it all in one
morning and a night, but then I did not
have *Mouth Music Made Easy*.

Happy heading.

This book is written as if you have never tried to go down on a woman before, which is ridiculous because you probably have. But this way we can cover all the bases. Your success rate may have been anything from abject failure to get to first nudge, all the way to having the neighbours call the cops to save the life of the screaming woman (it happens). So it's up to you to pick and choose from the following according to your own experience and her needs.

Let us assume you have already found a great love relationship or at the very least suspect you have. (Note: this is not a guide on 'how to pick up women' or any of that stuff; this is a guide to just one aspect of a sexual coupling.) You may have known her only a short time or have been married to her for fifteen years, or even fifty. The point is, you want to do something dazzling.

Why something dazzling? You need to ask? Is this the love of your life?

Here is a sad 'joke' told to me by a colleague with a growing pot belly and a wife he never stopped complaining about.

Question: What is the best way to give a woman an orgasm?

Answer: Who cares?

This man also once stated that a couple of nips of Scotch are more beneficial than sex and a lot less bother. He expected *me* to agree.

Is it a bit late for 'dazzling'? You never know. Dazzle her and she may dazzle you back.

Then again you may want to dazzle her for the same reason you send her flowers when it's *not* her birthday.

You'll have your own reason.

Let us also assume that you've done all
the preliminaries. You each have the
space and inclination. You've kissed,
touched, negotiated, fondled, danced to
the music, removed bits of clothing
(some of it, all of it, or if it's your thing,
put special items on), strewn rose petals
on the bed, cracked that bull whip a
couple of times for effect and rolled out
the bearskin.

You have eye contact, body contact,
hands touch and stroke and then, while
nibbling your ear, she says those words,
'Go down on me, I want oral sex, give me
a tongue lashing. Put your head between
my legs.'

Preliminaries should also include the
supply of a couple of fresh towels. Hand
towels will do. Some people use tissues
in the bedroom. Try using them to wipe
your wet chin and you'll see why a towel
is better. Toilet paper has no place
during sex. Ban it. And finally, shut
out all distractions. You know the drill.
Dazzle and distraction have little in
common except the letter 'D'.

Do you dread the word 'head'?

Or love it? Does your heart go ZING?

Does your belly go into a knot?

Do you break out in a sweat?

Do you know why?

Do you say 'Ah! Yes!'

or

'Oh? Um . . . Yeah. Well . . . OK? If you want to.'

Better you work this one out for yourself before you roll out the bearskin.

A surprising number of women think they 'smell funny down there'. If they think like that, is it any wonder some men get confused? Women do smell different. The top half smells of the deodorant, cosmetics, shampoo and perfume that mask all her natural identifying body scent; and the sex bit is right next to the plumbing. So you might be associating different with dangerous. And if we all did that the human race would have died out long ago.

Remember the first time you drank coffee? EECH! Or sneaked dad's beer as a kid? YUCK! You took a little time to acquire the taste. And there must have been other things you tried that seemed a bit unusual at first. See, you have had practice at acquiring a taste! You just need to get acclimatized.

Anticipate something new . . .

Anticipation is everything. Make her
wait. Work your way down slowly.
You're circling her nipples and nipping
at her belly, skirting the very edge of her
pubic area and giving butterfly kisses up
the insides of her thighs beginning
around her knees. You'll have your own
version(s) of this but you get the idea.
If she is *begging*, begging you to speed
up, you are probably about slow
enough. Be a little cruel. But if you
detect annoyance in her voice then
you're too slow. Speed up just a little.
Maybe a little more.

Giving head gives a man a sense
of power.

Ah! Cruelty! If you have not discovered
the joys of cruelty – nice cruelty –
this is a good time to get a little practice.
She knows what she wants, what she
thinks she requires, and you are going to
give it all to her – at a slower rate than
she expects. Not that you'll withhold
anything. Just slow it down. Let her
anticipate. Help her become more
sensitized. When her expectation is
running ahead of things it's like fine-
tuning an FM radio.

Naturally, once she's had this from you,
she might just do you the same dreadful
favour another time.

By now she should be in that classic
missionary position – on her back,
knees bent, thighs open – and you are
lying on your front, resting on your
elbows, between her legs. Make sure you
are *very* comfortable. You will be here
for a while. Don't crouch on your knees.
You'll get a crick in your neck. Your
discomfort could cost her an orgasm and
that's no way to win a friend and
influence the woman of your dreams.
If she is slightly built be certain to put
a pillow under her bottom to boost her
up. But make sure the pillow doesn't get
in your way. She's comfortable, you're
comfortable.

Ah! Yes!

You've made it this far and a certain, probably already familiar scent is presenting itself. If you love this aroma you can skip this page. But if you don't like it, what can be done?

First off, tell yourself this is not an unpleasant smell. Go on. It's not. It is a natural scent. You have one too and no matter how much you wash, it never quite goes away. It can be very sexy. If it's more than several hours since she had a shower her scent may be quite strong. You may also detect some urine smell on her pubic hair. She blots but some always remains. It will not harm you. Some health fanatics drink the stuff – they call it 'water of life'. Though I doubt the benefits it certainly doesn't kill them. There will also be normal sweat and, depending on her daily routine, perhaps a trace of faecal smell. Uh! Oh!

Hey! You're acclimatising.

One good way to begin is to blow gently on her pubic hair. These hairs, stiffer than ordinary hair, are attached to some very sensitive spots. Think of pubic hairs as the cat's whiskers. Your breath is very warm. And it will stir up her natural perfume.

As we humans evolved we reduced our body hair to a minimum. Science has concluded that the startling patch of prominent hair surrounding the genitals has been retained as a scent trap. You just opened the trap. Her female perfume floats straight up your male nose, across your male receptors and your male brain goes SNAP! A groan of genuine delight at this point will impress her beyond measure, as your brain shouts, 'Wow! Give me *more*.'

Some of us get really turned on by this heady combination. If it is too much for you, it is perfectly OK to ask her to come and have a shower (which has its own possibilities).

Or you could fetch a warm wet flannel and freshen her body for her as a part of your lovemaking. Remember soap irritates her sensitive bits and tastes awful. Minimize or eliminate it. Pat her dry with a fluffy towel. Her perfume will now be soft and gentle.

Male noses and male brains are programmed to respond. Yours will too. If you're a victim of an acquired negative attitude give yourself time. You might have to try this on a couple of occasions before your brain cells overcome those ancient playground jokes and go 'WOW!'

'Give me more!'

More could be using your fingers to
brush just the tips of her hair. You're
not ruffling. You are barely touching.
You can feel almost nothing yourself
but she can.

Now here is a problem some people have with pleasuring another. How do you know you are doing it right if you can't 'feel' much yourself? Some people might think, 'If I stick my cock in her watchyamacallit I know she must be feeling good because I am'.

BULLSHIT!

If this is you, change your mindset. Read on. You'll get the idea.

More could be delving in with your nose. Part her pubic hair right up the middle using your nose. That's good. Now how about parting her lovely cleft with the tip of your nose.

Sometimes a woman's inner vaginal lips begin to 'pout', to protrude as she becomes aroused. Go down there and find those beautiful lips. Take them between your own (when you are really skilful you can use your teeth but for heaven's sake, don't bite – don't even nibble – *caress*) and use the tip of your tongue to separate them. Play with them. Explore her lips using your lips and tongue.

Here comes our first Important Word.
There will be a few of these as we go
along. Remember them as a kind of
shorthand guide; it'll be easier than
having her read this book aloud to you
while you are trying to 'do the job'.

The first word is *EXPLORE*. Never cease
your exploration.

This nose-play and lip-play is simply
foreplay to giving head. You thought
oral sex was the foreplay? Think again.
For her, getting head is often *the* Main
Event – many women find it easier to
orgasm if there's clitoral stimulation.

That doesn't mean there can't be a
second Main Event.

And listen to her. Your lover may not be
talkative at this point in time, so listen
for the noises she makes. The little
sounds. Did you hear her catch her
breath? What precisely did you do to
cause that? Do it again. Did it work?
No? Let's try it again, three millimetres
over this way. She may move herself.
For you it will always be an exploration.
Remember that. Every time you do this
her body will feel different, react
differently. Not a lot. The sensitive
spots, those really magic ones, will move
around in subtle ways even she will not
be aware of. But you will. If you take
nothing for granted, take your time and
make every sexual occasion a fresh
exploration.

Second word: *LISTEN*.

Listen not just with your ears but with all your senses. Listen to the messages she is sending with her movements, taste, her body's changing texture, tension, heightening aroma. You name it. This is real body language. There are lots of little signals telling you how you are doing.

And there's that other word again: *EXPLORE*. And *LISTEN*. Apply them together.

Now you move the tip of your nose or perhaps the tip of your tongue, parting the folds, oh so very slowly, all the way to the top of her cleft.

Third word: *SLOWLY*.

Her area of operations is so small and so full of possibilities that you will miss so much by being too fast.

Think about it. If her tiny clit has as many nerve endings as your own cock then the possibilities within her vaginal cleft multiply out to the size of a football stadium.

Go *SLOWLY, EXPLORE, LISTEN*.

You've got it made.

Then there is the really advanced opener. For this you need to know each other really well and it's best she be fresh out of the shower. From your comfortable missionary position put your hands behind her knees and push her legs up, lifting her body so she is wholly exposed. Put your head and tongue as far down towards her back as you can reach and slide your tongue slowly forward. When you reach her anus circle right around it . . . then go slowly around it again and then ever so slowly explore your way all over it . . . before moving on up over the perineum (the bit in-between) to those pouting lips and then all the way to the top as you lower her back to the bed. You may have to pull her down from the ceiling.

Not ready for that one? That's OK.

But . . . if you want to give this a try and are a tad curious, try using lots of saliva on your tongue. And remember her anus is fresh and clean, cleaner than her feet, which have just walked from the bathroom – if you're a toe sucker.

Your anus gives you lots of pleasurable sensations doing nothing more than that which it was designed to do. Think fondly of yours. Pleasure hers.

All 'How To' books give lots of diagrams
so you can see what it is you are
supposed to be doing. This book is the
exception. What's the use of a picture if
you are working in the dark? The only
illustration of any use would have to be
in braille. Besides that, a picture is flat
and we are working very much in three
dimensions. Close your eyes and focus
on your other four senses – touch,
taste, smell and hearing. Never stop
listening to her small sounds.

There are plenty of book illustrations
out there with labels and arrows, if you
think you need them. But really, the
only diagram you require is herself.
Study it with your eyes closed.

As King Solomon said several thousand years ago, 'The joints of a woman's thighs are the work of a cunning workman.' By comparison, your penis is a blunt instrument.

Your tongue, however, dances around all day helping you talk, shout, sing, whistle, eat, drink, taste, chew, swallow, tell jokes and laugh at them, all the while avoiding your teeth. Versatile and clever, it qualifies as the perfect sexual partner.

Right now her perfect partner is resting somewhere near the top end of her lovely cleft. Do I hear a male brain shouting in your ear, 'That's where the clit is. Go for it, man. Go for it.' By all means have a gentle probe around but chances are it's in hiding. Leave it be. It'll ambush you later.

Yes, old King Solomon was right. And a
penis is a simple, dumb thing. Sure it
gives you pleasure but it ain't necessarily
giving her pleasure. As you really get to
know a female body you'll realize that
she does not so much receive pleasure
as take pleasure from a penis. Her bits
really get to work on your bit. Every
part of her cleft is interconnected and it
all moves and works in unison. This is
the work of a cunning work*man*. Her
genitals are the perfect pleasuring
device for a male. Women got second
best. God is definitely a fella.

Now . . . open your eyes for a moment and use your fingers to gently spread her upper cleft. Not too far. About a thumb width is plenty for now. This reveals her soft pink skin inside. As she becomes more aroused this pink colour will change to that of the crimson blush on a ripe peach or mango. Some women go quite purple. She never sees this but you will. Down here you will find out things about your lady that even she does not know. Allow your tongue to familiarize itself with this pink fold before you move back down to where you previously explored those luscious, pouting lips. You had a small taste of her juices the first time you moved your tongue along her cleft. It's time for you to become more familiar with them, to help her increase the flow and to put those juices to uses.

But steady on, remember your
three words:

Go *SLOWLY*

LISTEN intently

EXPLORE everything

A vagina is in some ways like your mouth. No, it doesn't have teeth! But it does have sensitive lips and, like your mouth, it is always wet. When you are hungry and smell food your mouth gets wetter. When a woman is sexually aroused her vagina gets wetter. Both are getting ready to receive. Mouths have saliva ducts, and vaginas have Bartholin's glands – named after the nineteenth-century doctor who was the first to describe them. (Let's not credit him with their 'discovery'. Fellas back then claimed to have discovered all sorts of new places that other people had been well aware of for centuries.) There are two of these little glands near the entrance to her vagina, plus another lubricating system further up. Their purpose is fairly obvious.

If you are having trouble getting used to the unusual taste and texture of her juice, dilute it with extra saliva. She, being already wet, will not notice what you are doing. Besides, you are giving her lots of pleasure.

And you are going to give her a great deal more.

It's this juice that gives a woman her
distinctive female smell. What does it
taste like? Try describing a wine vintage.
The nuance is individual and varies with
her menstrual cycle, state of health, what
she eats, drinks and so on. For instance,
smoking cigarettes will give a slight but
distinct bitter edge to her taste. But
generally speaking, and by my taste
buds, this is the land of milk and honey.
With an added dash of spice – sometimes
cinnamon, sometimes a trace of cayenne.
At the beginning it may be as thin as
champagne but as she become more and
more aroused it thickens, becomes
creamier, and by orgasm will have a rich
honey-like texture and consistency. No
chef ever presented a man with a better
dessert.

Work your tongue around her inner lips and tenderly begin to pull her further open with your hands. If she wants more she will no doubt be co-operating by opening her thighs wider, but use your hands anyway. Your hands are better than hers because you can easily change hand positions as necessary, while hers can sometimes get in your way. Peel her inner lips slowly open and run your tongue right down and around and into the entrance of her vagina.

Experiment with your hand positions.

Go slowly.

Explore.

Listen.

Explore some more . . . Slowly . . .

You are beginning to recognize shapes
and textures and tastes.

Now I take it we have all seen those
magazines and movies that show people
pretending to have wild sexual
encounters. Have you noticed that they
show penetrative sex between consenting
adults who somehow never seem to
touch one another? They invade each
other's body but not their personal
space. If you are one of the two per cent
who have managed to resist your
curiosity and never seen pornography
then that's OK. You will not have to
unlearn the following . . .

One thing is for certain, the Stud in the porno film never gets the part about those three Important Words.

Oh sure he can hear her going 'ooh, ooh, ooh' and making that sucking sound with her teeth. He knew it was coming; he read it in the script.

These movies always show oral sex
where the Stud has his tongue stuck
right out, skimming the general area of
the Actress's clit. The Stud has his head
rocked over on one side so the
cameraman can get his lens in (it's called
a 'pull back'), and so he can keep one
eye on the cameraman to be sure his
best profile is being filmed.

If you do it that way you'll get a
sore tongue and she'll be a
disappointed woman.

Oh! No!

It is really not a good idea to stick your tongue out and put it on her genitals. Neither is it much use sticking your tongue into her genitals. To achieve your mutual aim of great oral sex you will have lovingly peeled her lips apart and placed your open mouth right down over her open mouth. You have, in effect, put her genitals right into your mouth. This is like tongue kissing with only one tongue.

Maximize contact. Your lower lip is
against the inside of her inner lips. Your
upper lip is on the lining of her upper
lips near her clit or just above it.
Everything feels incredibly smooth. Your
tongue is opposite the entrance of her
vagina. If you push your tongue forward
about as far as you would if you were
normally wetting your lips you will
make effortless, tireless, sustained
contact.

You have reached the launch pad. Now
you send her into orbit.

CONTACT!

If necessary use your hands to open her
that little bit more so you can get that
lower lip into position. Your lower lip
can be almost as effective as your
tongue. Try it.

From now on never break contact with those sensitive parts. You have a tongue, lips, fingers. It's important that an uninterrupted flow of sensations be travelling up her body. Your tongue is sliding around her vaginal entrance and pretty soon, if not already, her ever-present juices will begin to flow. And I mean *really* flow. Take your time. Take your cues from her. Go slowly. It will happen. You will get that tongueful of rich juice. Ah, here it comes. Savour it. Now get some of that juice and scoop it up along her cleft to her clit or the place where her clit soon will appear. Scoop lots of it up.

As things progress, go back every couple of minutes for another scoop. Keep her clit slick and lubricated.

If you are producing lots of saliva and need to swallow, you can disguise your swallow by sliding that lower lip up or with some other ploy such as a series of little kisses in the same area where your tongue has been in action. You may, of course, choose not to swallow and simply let your saliva flow – she really won't notice the extra wetness and this way you will maintain maximum contact with her pleasure parts.

Theory: There is something in a woman's juices that has a direct effect on her clitoris. Something about her sweet liquid makes her clit swell beautifully and become more sensitive. Maybe this is a chemical reaction. Maybe it's to do with the very slippery texture. Anyway, it works.

Now we have a fourth word: *SCOOP*.

Now I don't know what you were taught
about sexual anatomy but I was taught
that the clitoris is this tiny little button
that if you could only find it and rub it
she would love you forever. When I
finally did find one it promptly went
back into hiding and the owner said,
'Ouch!' All I did was rub it like I
was told.

In fact she levitated. But not in the way
I had intended.

Beware of where you picked up your
knowledge. Even after years of
experience you might still have the
wrong idea about one or two things.
Be open to fresh information.

Recent medical research, although not yet conclusive, indicates why there's more to giving head to a woman than sticking out your tongue. Although not conclusive, if you act as though it is, you will both get very satisfactory results.

First, while it's true that the entire human body is an erogenous zone, within her body a woman has two major sexually sensitive spots. They are the clitoris and the G spot. The clit is the little button at the top of the cleft near the urethra. The G spot is a spongy mound just up in the vagina on the front wall, roughly the distance from your fingertip to the second knuckle.

Second, stop thinking of them as two spots and pretend they are one.

So, having told you to beware of
unfounded information, here I am
giving you unfounded information.

Give it a try anyway. This works.

Read on.

It makes sense. Nature uses the same systems over and over again. Men and women become sexually aroused in much the same way using blood flow and erectile tissue. Our faces and chests flush, our eyes dilate, our nipples become erect and our genitals swell in much the same way.

In fact, erectile tissue occurs all over the human body, even in your nose. (Keep breathing, man.) Your lips swell when there is delicious food around – or when you are kissing your lover – but probably not when you're kissing great-auntie Maud.

Nothing new here.

Keep scooping.

So, without going into too much detail,
think of her anatomy in similar terms as
your own. You understand your own.
Her vaginal lips are like your scrotum.
When you caress or suck on her lips,
imagine what she is feeling is something
like what you get when she touches you
down there. (And remember the
difference between a touch and an
attack.) The base of your penis is
attached just in front of your anus.
So is her G spot. What you get when
she touches the very base of your cock
is what she gets when you touch her
G spot. The button we think of as the
clit is like the tip of your penis and in
between her clit and G spot think of a
structure very much like your own cock
buried in the vaginal wall.

Watch out!

There's a whole bunch of writers on sexuality who have built careers on the question: *'Why do men act as if women's bodies respond sexually in the same way as male bodies? Women are different!'* They go on to explain why this is so, and will probably disagree with what I have written in the next few pages. We know that her emotions can be different, and that her body is different, but what physical sensations is she having? How can you do this thing to her satisfaction if you don't know that? It's like teaching a fish to fly.

The comparisons I am asking you to make between the male and female bodies are merely translations. There is a chance they could be wildly wrong but they are the best information we are likely to have – and they work for me. So give the translations a go.

Think of her clit as being about a third
of the length of your cock, thick at the
base, tapering rapidly to a point and
shaped something like a clove of garlic.
This isn't a penis. It is still a clitoris. It is
just a bit bigger than we were led to
believe and it burrows right through her.

And . . .

It gets just as aroused and erect as
you do.

Make love to her clitoris as if it were
your own. Caress it up. Make it erect.
Pretend you are her doing this to you.
What would you like? How does she get
you erect? Work the underside of her
clitoris, which is exposed within her
opened cleft. You know exactly how to
do this. Remember to use her natural
lubricant. Scoop it up. Her clit has the
same number of nerve endings as your
penis, but in a smaller area. It's extremely
sensitive, maybe as sensitive to pain as a
testicle. Keep that in mind. It's always
better to start too gentle. She'll soon let
you know. And again the emphasis is on
exploration. Tongue pressure that took
her to screaming ecstasy last time may
make her just scream this time. Go easy.
Go slowly. Build it up. Every time is a
new exploration.

As you explore, vary what you do with your tongue. Use your tongue pressed flat against her or edge-on deep in her groove. The underside of your tongue has a different texture to the top, so try using that too. Push the tip up under her hood but watch the pressure. Remember your tongue is a muscle and quite strong.

And keep that clitoris slick with juice. Scoop every few minutes.

And there you are. She is swelling up
tighter and tighter. She is getting wetter
and wetter, creamier and creamier. If she
is about to come, don't change a thing.
She may move slightly if she needs to
fine-tune what you are doing but you
stay with what you are doing. This is
not the time for big changes.

As the big moment draws closer she
may even start to move around quite
a lot. Her whole pelvis could begin
jumping about. Try not to break
contact. Ride it out.

(Try keeping your tongue and lips fixed
in exactly the same spot while she is
jumping about. You won't succeed but
it's fun to try and can be very rewarding.)

'Wait a minute. What if she farts?' asks that timid male brain of yours. 'Don't women sometimes fart when they come? Isn't this going to be a big orgasm? Look where my nose is.'

Don't worry. Your nose is well out of the firing line so chin down, mind on the job.

'What if she pees?' No big deal. Some women pee a little at climax. It's perfectly clean when fresh and no danger to man or beast. If it happens, dilute with useful extra saliva.

If she is not there yet you could add an
extra dimension. Move one hand so that
your thumb and index finger are
holding her open. Slide a finger from
your other hand up into her vagina
(wet it first, there's plenty of juice) and
caress that G spot. Again, imagine what
it's like when she is giving you head and
fondles the very base of your soon to
explode cock.

Oh! Yes!

Or she might sometimes need your finger further inside. An orgasm is a series of contractions that quiver right down her vagina. Her vagina might need to have something to grip or resist against to intensify the contractions. This might happen sometimes, every time or never. If she doesn't already know she won't find out if *you* don't explore the possibilities . . .

SLOWLY.

Careful with the fingernails.

Again, sometimes, every time or never, she might like anal stimulation. I don't mean jamming your finger into her. Maybe a gentle fingertip external exploration is what she needs. Or maybe just a little pressure using the pad of your thumb – like the hint of a promise of penetration. If she does want finger penetration let her tell you. Wet your finger with her juices and go gently. But this is a sometimes-sensitive area of sexuality so it is best not to take too much initiative. Ask her afterwards, 'Would you have preferred if I had . . .' Or say, 'I really wanted to . . .' But don't ask her now. She's busy.

And remember, these are extras, not the main game. Don't forget your lips and your tongue.

So there you are, flying solo, so to speak. You have her neatly at the brink. Here is one last piece of advice. We men tend to like things hard and fast. Not all of us but that's the tendency. Don't assume that she wants the same. I've been saying all along you should err on the soft and gentle side. Now she is getting near the end don't fall into the trap of speeding up. Just because what you are doing is working, do not think that doing it harder and faster is going to be better. It may be for you and it may even be for her but don't assume. Try slowing right down. Same thing only slower. Do not increase the pressure unless she indicates that you should. Edge her toward the precipice. Faster is always less accurate. It is not a race.

Is dinner tastier if eaten fast?

listen

slowly

listen

slowly

slowly!

keep exploring

it's not a race . . .

She's nearly there. All your senses tell
you what you want to know. Your
hearing tells you that her breathing has
changed, she may be whispering things
she won't remember afterwards, your
taste buds are flooded with her juices,
nose assailed with pheromones, her
body is jumping and quivering with
pleasure . . .

And then everything stops. You think
'Oh! NO! She's lost it. Where did it go?
What did I do wrong?' The only thing
you did wrong was to stop now. This is
the calm before the storm. The eye of
the cyclone. Keep going.

DON'T CHANGE A THING.

I'll step out now. It's six seconds to
ground zero.

No rush.

When you're ready.

Wipe your chin. There's a towel beside you. And she may need one to put over the wet spot. Between your saliva and her juices there's quite a deal of liquid here. Did she come?

Yes? Wonderful.

No? Keep exploring. Next time, maybe. The point is . . . you still *pleasured* her.

Once you get rid of any negative attitudes you might have had and overcome her apprehensions – 'Are you sure I don't smell funny?' 'Do you really like doing that?' – and learn to revel in her, you cannot help but to reassure and *pleasure* the lady . . . and this in turn can give rise to some very un*lady*like orgasms in future. One day maybe your neighbours will call the emergency services.

'But,' you might ask, 'haven't we missed something?'

And you'd be right. We have concentrated entirely on oral sex as Main Event. I've given specific instructions on really only one position and, while this position is enormously useful for long and tireless devouring, I've left out all those imaginative hors d'oeuvres and surprises you will no doubt encounter as you become more experienced. Be she standing, squatting or kneeling, give your head any way it will fit. Do what feels good.

But what the long, slow, comfortable method does superbly is give you a feel for what you are doing, a way to get to know her sexual anatomy as no book, no matter how well illustrated, can ever teach you. And getting that feel for her now can only lead to tastier hors d'oeuvres and lovelier surprises in times to come.

LISTEN
   EXPLORE
      SLOWLY
        SCOOP

And love her while you devour her.
Good sex always was and forever will be
much more than technique.

Read the book again and learn to do
every bit. It's like playing music. You
learn every note of the score, decide how
each note is to be played – pressed,
plucked, stroked – put together the
phrases, the melodies, the rhythms,
practise till you know it backwards and
then . . . forget it all . . . and just play
the music.

Play well.

PAY OFF

Yes, there is a pay off. For one thing you should have a very happy woman sharing your life. That is always good.

What you have after giving skilled head is a woman swollen with pleasure, flushed, erect, purple with desire and wanting your candybar. As you increase your skills her body will come to expect increasing quantities of pleasure and get still more tight and wet in anticipation. You may find she is so swollen after oral sex that you have trouble getting inside. Don't worry. There's lots of her fragrant juice to help you out. Or should that be in . . .

Prepare to be *dazzled*.

Listen, you will never *explore* to the end of her. Be on the lookout, there will always be something new to learn. *Scoop* the juice, go *slowly* and you won't miss out.

Play that mouth music.

HOT SEX
How to do it
by Tracey Cox

'Tracey Cox is stunningly well informed about sex. She can tell a G-spot from an A-spot and could probably find both of them before the rest of us have got the map references'
The Mirror

Practical, down to earth, explicit and fun, *Hot Sex* is the must-have sex and relationships book for every woman and man.

It's perfect bedtime reading for two, an easy-to-follow guide that cuts straight to the nitty gritty to deliver candid advice with a healthy dose of humour. Packed with tips and techniques that work, *Hot Sex* includes everything from a blow-by-blow, step-by-step guide to oral sex to finding (and figuring out) your G-spot.

Whether you're a beginner or an old hand, get into *Hot Sex* – the only how-to that really tells you how to do it!

'What distinguishes Cox is at the heart of her appeal: the ability to talk about sex in a universal way'
The Times

'A brilliant book to get hold of if you're planning a night in with the girls'
Woman's Own

0 552 14707 9

THE GOOD GIRL'S GUIDE TO BAD GIRL SEX
An Indispensable Guide to Pleasure and Seduction
by Barbara Keesling Ph.D.

Imagine a world where you were as sexually confident, physically uninhibited and intensely orgasmic as you have always wanted to be . .

Now, acclaimed sex therapist Dr Barbara Keesling tells you how. Based on the understanding that inside every good girl is a bad girl struggling to get out, *The Good Girl's Guide to Bad Girl Sex* teaches women how to express their natural impulses with dignity and panache. Bad girls know no shame. Bad girls are comfortable in their bodies. Bad girls always feel gorgeous and desirable!

Learn how to optimize your sexual power with this frank, funny and thoroughly comprehensive book. Packed with practical exercises, *The Good Girl's Guide* includes insider information on the sex toys you never knew you had, how to seduce a man by simply walking into a room, how to enjoy your G-spot and how to give (and receive!) mind-blowing orgasms.

The Good Girl's Guide is the key to your sexual future – an invaluable resource for the modern woman.

A Bantam Paperback

0 553 81475 3

302 ADVANCED TECHNIQUES FOR DRIVING A MAN WILD IN BED
by Olivia St. Claire

The author of the hugely successful and perennially popular, *203 Ways to Drive a Man Wild in Bed* is back with an all-new, easy-to-use guide that elevates sexual proficiency and erotic ecstasy to an entirely new level.

'The secret lies not in comeliness or technique, but in the fearlessness to reveal your truest female self', writes Olivia St. Claire as she refines the art of driving him wild. Olivia helps you identify your passion triggers, safely guides you to the edge of your boundaries, and tells you everything you ever wanted to know about truly passionate lovemaking.

Frankly erotic, playfully sexy and intelligently written, *302 Advanced Techniques for Driving a Man Wild in Bed* is simple enough to consult at a moment's notice, but sophisticated enough to leave him breathless at your new-found prowess. The inviting layout and the numbered tips make it easy and fun for a willing couple to embark upon an amorous adventure – whenever and wherever the spirit moves them. Users of this dazzling selection of sexual techniques will bring any man to his knees.

A Bantam paperback

0 553 81473 7

A SELECTION OF NON-FICTION TITLES AVAILABLE
FROM CORGI AND BANTAM BOOKS

THE PRICES SHOWN BELOW WERE CORRECT AT THE TIME OF GOING TO PRESS.
HOWEVER TRANSWORLD PUBLISHERS RESERVE THE RIGHT TO SHOW NEW
RETAIL PRICES ON COVERS WHICH MAY DIFFER FROM THOSE PREVIOUSLY
ADVERTISED IN THE TEXT OR ELSEWHERE.

99845 1	THE NEW ASTROLOGY FOR WOMEN		
		Jessica Adams	£9.99
09806 X	WHAT DO YOU SAY AFTER YOU SAY HELLO?		
		Eric Berne M.D.	£5.99
81354 4	THE BOOK OF ANSWERS	*Carol Bolt*	£9.99
81487 7	THE BOOK OF LOVE ANSWERS	*Carol Bolt*	£9.99
14707 9	HOT SEX	*Tracey Cox*	£7.99
14784 2	HOT RELATIONSHIPS	*Tracey Cox*	£7.99
14956 X	HOT SEX POCKET EDITION	*Tracey Cox*	£4.99
14955 1	HOT LOVE POCKET EDITION	*Tracey Cox*	£4.99
14938 1	THE FABULOUS GIRL'S GUIDE TO DECORUM		
		Kim Izzo & Ceri	£6.99
81496 6	ZEN AND THE ART OF FALLING IN LOVE		
		Charlotte Kasl	£6.99
81475 3	THE GOOD GIRL'S GUIDE TO BAD GIRL SEX		
		Barbara Keesling	£6.99
15025 8	I WAS A TEENAGE DOMINATRIX	*Shawna Kenney*	£5.99
81371 4	LIFE MAKEOVERS	*Cheryl Richardson*	£7.00
50473 8	203 WAYS TO DRIVE A MAN WILD IN BED		
		Olivia St. Claire	£5.99
50485 1	227 WAYS TO UNLEASH THE SEX GODDESS IN EVERY WOMAN	*Olivia St. Claire*	£6.99
81473 7	302 ADVANCED TECHNIQUES FOR DRIVING A MAN WILD IN BED	*Olivia St. Claire*	£6.99
81488 5	THE ORACLE BOOK	*Georgia Routsis Savas*	£9.99
40397 4	THE FRAGRANT PHARMACY	*Valerie Ann Worwood*	£5.99

All Transworld titles are available by post from:

Bookpost, PO Box 29, Douglas, Isle of Man, IM99 1BQ

Credit cards accepted. Please telephone 01624 836000
fax 01624 837033, Internet http://www.bookpost.co.uk
or e-mail: bookshop@enterprise.net for details

**Free postage and packing in the UK. Overseas customers: allow £1 per book
(paperbacks) and £3 per book (hardbacks)**